WHO TAKES CARE OF THE CARETAKER?

Taking Your Life Back

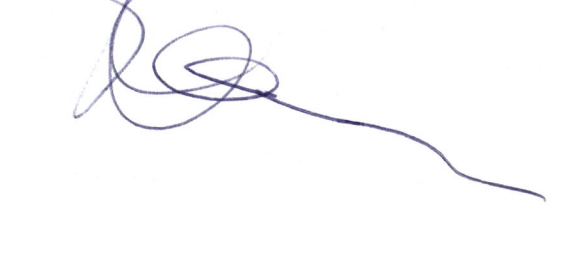

Tom Krause

© 2016 Tom Krause
All rights reserved.

ISBN: 1539604039
ISBN 13: 9781539604037

Thank you, Vivian York Williamson.

Every person needs a caring, nurturing, encouraging friend.

Dedicated to all caretakers who make the world a better place.

The Caretaker's Creed

It only takes a moment
to reach out to be a friend,
but to the one who needs you,
the memory never ends.

A simple act of kindness
to a person you don't know
may plant a seed of friendship
that for them will always grow.

We sometimes lose perspective
on the difference we can make
when we care more for our giving
and care less for what we take.

So remember that your actions
may help change a life someday.
Always think about the person
that you meet along your way.

For it only takes a moment
to reach out to be a friend,
but to the one who needs you,
the memory never ends.

INTRODUCTION

Hey you!
Are you a caretaker?
Do people expect everything from you?
Are you tired? Stressed? Overwhelmed?
Expectations, responsibilities, expectations, responsibilities?

Do you feel like all your time and energy is being used up in caring for others, leaving little for yourself?

Do you feel frustrated, hurt, disrespected, or invisible when it comes to people caring for your needs in return?

Is caretaking ruining your health? Is it ruining your relationships with others? Is it making you not like yourself? Do you feel as if you have no control?

Do you ever wonder *who takes care of the caretaker*?

What is a Caretaker?

Think for a moment before you get busy today
of the nicest person you have met on life's way—
how accepted you felt, the interest they showed.
So happy to see you. A smile that just glowed.
You could talk of your dreams, share stories and jokes.
You could share your concerns and worries and hopes.
Words of support were all you received.
Encouraging thoughts that helped you believe.
And not for a moment did you ever feel judged.
You could be who you were. You always felt loved.
You see, the happiest people have hearts full of love.
They are humble and thankful for gifts from above.
They make others feel special for they believe
that they are.
They have struggled in life but have covered
their scars.
Contentment they've found from not thinking
of self.
God has taught them the joy of loving
somebody else.
Now think for a moment as you start on your way:
wouldn't it be nice to be that person today?

What I have just described is a caretaker—a wonderful person most of us would like to model ourselves after, a person who filled our lives with precious memories of how we were accepted, how we were believed in, and how we were loved.

This book is about recognizing and appreciating caretakers. It is about how to help these wonderful souls deal with the everyday stresses that come from being a caretaker. Most of all, it is about how to care for those who care for us.

CHAPTER 1
WHO ARE CARETAKERS?

Some people are caretakers by nature. They possess very dominant qualities of nurturing and love. They see other people through humanistic eyes, almost feeling their emotions with them.

Caretakers are easily drawn into situations involving relationships where they feel the need to help. Whether at work or at home, caretakers are driven to make sure people are cared for in their time of need.

While this motivation is admirable, eventually it simply becomes too stressful, too painful, or too exhausting. No person is superhuman. Caretaker also have needs that must be met. It can affect their physical and mental health if they are not. In those situations this question needs to be asked: Who takes care of the caretaker?

By definition, caretakers are people who give care to somebody or something. For our purposes in this book, caretakers are people who are passionate about taking care of people in need. They may also be known as caregivers. Unlike those who serve others out of selfish reasons for their own gain, true caretakers see caring for their fellow man as a life purpose that they gladly undertake. There is a humbleness and peace about serving others that fill their soul. Other people may not understand. There are takers and caretakers in this world. A taker dies with an empty heart; a caretaker's heart is full.

Caretakers are blessed and cursed with a righteous soul. They hurt when others hurt. They do not like unfairness or injustice. They worry for loved ones when the world treats them cruelly. Caretakers may remain silent when they are treated badly, but they will be the first to stand up and speak out for others. They are more apt to get in trouble by defending someone else than by defending themselves. They are led by their spirit to encourage, comfort, defend, and guide people in their lives. They teach people they care for to get up when they fall down. While they are not actually angels with wings, they are sometimes equated to human angels who are sent to perform very similar angelic tasks.

Caretakers become the gatekeepers for those they care for, both physically and emotionally. They do not let bad influences around them. They take responsibility for what happens on their watch to their loved ones. They teach right from wrong to their children. They nurture spiritual and moral values.

My father was a caretaker. He was quiet man who taught us by the way he lived. Though he passed away many years ago, his example of gatekeeping for the children he cared for still stands out in my mind today. While the world may not be fair, in my father's house, people were treated with fairness. While the world may be full of entitlement, in my father's house, people were treated equally. While the world may have mocked, ridiculed, or treated some badly, in my father's house, people were treated with respect. By his actions, we learned that, even though the whole world may become hopeless, in his house we would always be hopeful.

My father taught us that each one of us can determine what we let into our house. Each of us can become the gatekeeper of what we allow around us. No matter "the way of the world," we all can make a choice of what is seen, what is heard, and what is tolerated by ourselves and our children. It may be true that one person cannot change the whole world, but individually, each person in his or her own way can make a difference.

Too much caretaking drains people of energy emotionally, physically, and in some cases financially. The more they give, the more they become expected to give. Others may not see the need to help because they have become dependent on the caretaker's coming to their rescue. Since caretakers by nature have to give, they become vulnerable to those who only want to take.

Caretakers, like most people, suffer from what we fail to do anything about. They never seem to have enough time get things done for themselves. There just aren't enough hours in the day free for their needs. Things keep being added to their plates, while nothing is ever taken off. They fall into the trap of living their lives in survival mode, serving others rather than self-satisfaction.

In today's world the use of antidepressant and antianxiety medication is soaring, and alcohol and illegal drug usage continues to destroy lives. Stress today, especially for caring people, is a very real problem.

While there are many medications available today to help caretakers cope with stress in their lives, sometimes pills are not enough. Even with these medications, caretakers need something more to help them cope with their hectic schedules. Hopefully, this book will help.

While no one can ever take all the stress out of life, there are ways to get some sort of handle on it. Maybe it can be made more manageable. Maybe some stress can even be eliminated. Only then can a caretaker like you take your life back so that you can move toward more happiness.

This book is about helping caretakers get their lives back by learning about stress and how to deal with it. It will focus on a specific type of stress that caring people especially encounter, as well as how too much stress affects not only physical health but mental health. It will look at how people with different personality types affect caretakers. Finally, the book will include a list of twenty-six coping skills designed to help caretakers manage the unavoidable stressors of daily life.

CHAPTER 2
CARETAKERS AND STRESS

Life becomes something we plow through. Most of us don't give ourselves enough credit for what we handle on a daily basis. Taking time to assess the stresses you deal with during any particular period of time may help you realize just how much stress you are really dealing with.

After I turned fifty-five years old, the following happened to me within five years: retirement, a cancer diagnosis, a stepson in a car accident in which four teenagers were killed, a separation, a divorce, a move, becoming a single parent, a change in financial status, starting a new career, and beginning a new relationship with a woman who still had a child at home.

Who Takes Care of the Caretaker?

Stress is the body's reaction to the world around you. The more demands we encounter in our daily lives, the more our stress increases. Even events we see as positive may add to a person's stress level.

Everyone deals with stress. A little stress is healthy. It motivates us to get things done. However, too much stress turns into distress, which can have corrosive, devastating effects on us over time.

Each person reacts to stress in his or her own way. What may be very stressful for one person may not faze another person. It is important to know yourself when it comes to what bothers you. Specific things that cause you stress are called *stressors*. The best way to identify the stressors in your life is to sit down and make a list of things currently causing you stress.

While you are at it, list how long you have been dealing with those stressors and any physical or emotional symptoms you have noticed in yourself as a result. If you haven't noticed any, consult people around you for their opinions. It is sometimes hard to see outside ourselves. Ask them to be honest about any changes they have noticed in your behavior. Don't compare your list with anyone else's; it is only how something affects *you* that is important.

As a caretaker, you may find stressors on your list that you have been dealing with for a long time. If you do, you may be suffering from a certain type of stress known as *chronic stress.*

Chronic stress is the kind of stress that arises out of long-lasting circumstances or events that you can't control. The circumstances or events may include but are not limited to the following:

- Being overwhelmed by the needs of others in a relationship.
- Feeling as if you have no help or support.
- Caring for someone with a significant illness or disability.
- Never having time to care for self needs or rest.
- Multiple significant losses over a period of time.

Chronic stress is a type of stress that caretakers are exposed to over an extended period of time. There is no break from this form of stress. It becomes a constant companion of the caregiver, slowly but surely breaking down their physical and emotional well-being.

Chronic stress affects a person's health by raising blood pressure, increasing the risk of stroke or heart attack, decreasing the immune system's effectiveness, and making the person more vulnerable to illness. It can also lead to increased anxiety as well as depression.

Stretch both of your arms out in front of you, and then make a fist with each hand at the same time. Now continue to squeeze both fists as tightly as you can for as long as you can. Eventually, you will tire and have to stop. As you open your hands, feel the pain in your fingers until they finally relax to their normal state of flexibility. Living with chronic stress is as if all of your body systems are being squeezed tight for years. The constant tension will eventually lead to fatigue. You will begin to experience pain in different parts of your body. For years your body has never been allowed to get back to its normal state of relaxation. Are you starting to get the picture?

Off-the-cuff comments like "My life is killing me" or "Stress has aged you" are actually true. I am always amazed by the way the physical appearance of those we've elected president of the United States changes from the time they enter office until they leave. Go back to look at before-and-after photos to see how much some of our most recent inhabitants of the Oval Office have aged during their terms. While we may not see our lives as being as stressful as the president's, the effects of chronic stress on us are the same. The only difference is that most of us don't have a team of doctors following us around, monitoring our health. We are left to monitor ourselves.

The tricky part of chronic stress is that sufferers get accustomed to it. Some caregivers have lived with the chronic stress of caring for people for so long that they believe what they are feeling is normal. Resolving oneself to chronic stress does not make the effects on health go away. Eventually symptoms grow worse.

CHAPTER 3
EFFECTS OF CHRONIC STRESS ON CARETAKERS

Legendary basketball coach Bobby Knight once said, "What you live with when you are winning, you die with when you are losing." I don't know if he was the first one to say that, but it is true. Problems that are ignored do not go away. The effects of chronic stress on caregivers are very real. These effects can be ignored for a while, but eventually they must be addressed. *Life isn't about living without problems. Life is about solving problems.*

Here is a composite list of the effects of chronic stress. See if any sound like something you've experienced:

- Headaches
- Body aches and pain
- Eating too much or too little
- Disturbed sleep
- Mood swings
- An urge to get away
- Irritability
- Constipation
- High blood pressure
- Weight gain
- Fatigue
- Poor concentration
- Forgetting things
- Increase in alcohol or tobacco consumption
- Irregular periods or loss of periods in women
- Claustrophobia

All these signs, if ignored, can lead to some very serious physical health issues, such as stroke, hypertension, depression, eating disorders, substance abuse, and insomnia, to name a few.

That does not even take into consideration how stress affects your mental health or your relationship with coworkers, family, and friends, which can be even more damaging.

Who Takes Care of the Caretaker?

Mental health has been defined as how you like, accept, and feel about yourself; how you relate to others; and how you meet the daily demands of life. People in good mental health are able to avoid having the demands of life overwhelm them.

Too much stress inhibits a person's ability to think clearly. Anxiety levels rise, causing difficulty in dealing with emotions such as anger or sadness in calm, logical ways. A tendency to overreact to normal emotional issues occurs, leading to verbal outbursts, aggressive behavior, and in some cases depression.

Caretakers and Fatigue

The greatest effect of chronic stress on caretakers is from fatigue—mental and physical fatigue caused by too much worry. Caregivers with high levels of worry become emotionally spent, with little tolerance or energy for themselves and others. They become quickly irritated with less patience for those around them.

The definition of worry is giving way to anxiety or unease or allowing one's mind to dwell on difficulty or troubles. It is usually caused by focusing too much on negative thoughts of what might occur in the future, rather than dealing with the realities of the present. Worry about loved ones, demands, and deadlines takes its toll on energy levels and produces physical, pathological, and psychological fatigue.

Physical fatigue is a feeling of tiredness or exhaustion caused by too much physical use of the muscles of the body, causing the body to need rest to regain energy. Pathological fatigue occurs from too much stress on the body's defense mechanisms fighting disease. Medicines and rest are usually the cure for pathological fatigue. Psychological fatigue is the feeling of tiredness and exhaustion caused by worry and stress. Unlike fatigue caused by too much physical exertion or the breakdown of the body's defenses to prevent disease, medicines and rest will not cure psychological fatigue caused by too much worry. The caretaker could sleep for hours, only to discover that he or she still feels exhausted after awakening. That is because the source of the person's worry still exists. Fatigue caused by worry cannot be eliminated until that which is causing the worry has been resolved. Only then does energy return.

Fatigue from stress left unchecked too long can lead to a diagnosis of chronic fatigue syndrome. Symptoms include the following:

Who Takes Care of the Caretaker?

- Persistent, severe fatigue for at least six months
- Mild fever and sore throat
- Headaches and joint pains
- Muscle weakness and pain
- Sleep problems
- Difficulty thinking clearly
- Fatigue after light exercise

All of the reasons above should be enough to quit ignoring a problem that is eating away at overstressed caregivers from within. The key point again is that chronic stress is a real problem. Real problems have real solutions, but problems don't get solved unless they are recognized and addressed. Refer to the coping skills in the last chapter for ways to reduce stress, worry, and fatigue. If that doesn't work, consult a physician. Don't just suffer in silence.

CHAPTER 4
CARETAKER HAVE NEEDS

As stated before, caretakers are much attuned to the needs of others, sometimes to the expense of their own. These are the needs caretakers see in others but often overlook in themselves. What caretakers need to be reminded of is that they have the same needs that must be met.

American psychologist Abraham Maslow theorized that human beings must meet certain needs inherent in all of us in order to achieve self-fulfillment (true happiness). Some needs are more powerful than others, and thus they must be satisfied first before other needs can be met. He listed these needs in the shape of a pyramid, placing the needs in order of priority from bottom to top. The following is a list of Maslow's hierarchy of needs.

Physical needs are our basic, most powerful needs. Our need to satisfy hunger and thirst, our need for sleep, and our need to feel safe, secure, and out of danger dominate our every thought. Just try to study when you are hungry or lacking sleep. It is possible, but the constant reminder of the need for food or sleep will keep slipping into your brain until it is satisfied.

Most people don't believe stealing is moral, but if they were hungry enough they would more than likely steal food to eat. Meeting these needs is essential. There is no need to go any further when it comes to self-fulfillment until these needs are satisfied. They are a constant concern to our well-being.

Since these needs are so powerful, people have no choice but to pay attention to them. They may try to skip meals or go with little sleep, but they soon learn that work suffers.

Emotional needs such as the need to love and be loved, the need to belong, and the need to feel worthwhile are next on the pyramid in terms of importance. Emotional needs are so critical that they can actually affect our physical health. Studies have shown that babies who are not picked up, held, or talked to can become physically and emotionally stunted. Their health deteriorates. In some cases, they can actually die from loneliness.

People who suffer from depression often describe their feelings as loneliness, lack of self-worth, and sadness. Children who are made fun of or picked on at school sometimes commit suicide. That is why being aware of the hurt from name-calling or bullying is very important.

The need to be valued and recognized is so powerful that people will go to great lengths to find acceptance. Emotional needs are why we have family and friends. In every person's life there needs to be a caring, nurturing, encouraging friend. People who validate our existence with common interests make us feel normal. In the case of loved ones, we feel loved and accepted.

Meeting our emotional needs is almost as important as eating and sleeping. It is not something to be taken lightly or ignored, yet caretakers too often tend to put their own emotional needs on the back burner. Slowly their mental health declines as their relationships with others suffer.

Aesthetic needs come into play when physical and emotional needs are met. People start to look outward from themselves to explore and appreciate the world around them, much like an infant who is fed and nurtured begins to discover his or her new life with all its wonders. The child becomes curious. He or she explores and searches for answers—and then begins to appreciate the beauty of the world. This is really the level where education takes place.

Struggling schools may recognize the importance of providing for the basic physical needs of their students. They may work hard to provide a safe, secure environment and to provide nutritious meals for their students. They provide classrooms filled with curricula to study.

However, what successful schools realize and struggling schools do not is that they must also provide an environment that recognizes and values children—a place where every child feels that he or she belongs. That is where caring, dedicated teachers make the most impact. When these emotional needs are met, students are ready to look outside themselves and learn.

With adults it is the same. Reaching this level provides us an understanding of the world outside our own. It expands our horizons, making us more well-rounded people.

Self-fulfilling needs are at the stage in which people self-actualize. They realize they are not only a member of the world, but they want to find ways to make a difference in the lives around them. Caretakers at this level find their purpose not only in caring for themselves but in reaching out to others. This is where life gets its meaning. Self-actualized people start to answer this question: "Why am I here?" A person who reaches this level starts to feel satisfied, complete, and self-fulfilled. People on this level finally find the happiness in life that they've been seeking.

Caretakers who completely put the needs of others above their own needs suffer the consequences. Physical illness, mental illness, or both may occur.

A caretaker's health suffers when he or she ignores such basic needs as rest, sleep, and proper diet. Caretakers' self-esteem suffers when they begin to feel taken for granted or when their own need to be valued and recognized goes ignored. Often, caretakers will spend so much time being concerned about others that they don't take time to discover or enjoy new things, and thus they don't fulfill their own aesthetic needs. Most importantly, when caretakers ignore their own needs, they may never reach the level of self-fulfillment that brings true happiness.

As a consequence, they begin to feel doomed to an existence that consists only of giving, without receiving anything in return.

CHAPTER 5
CARETAKERS' EMOTIONS

Caretakers take on the feelings of others. When someone they care for feels emotions, they are likely to feel the same emotions. Just as parents worry when their children are not happy, all caregivers worry about the people they are caring for. Dealing with this type of emotional relationship can be very draining.

Love and Guilt

When caretakers love someone, they feel the need to truly do all they can to show their love for that person. Because they are so attuned to the emotional needs of the ones they care for, they can also feel guilt when they sense they are not meeting the needs or expectations of their loved ones. It is human nature to seek out acceptance. Caretakers want to feel acceptance from the one they love. An unhealthy way to find acceptance is to become a *people pleaser*.

When a caretaker falls into the people-pleaser trap, they mistakenly believe that the only way to find acceptance is to make others like them. Their need to please others becomes an endless endeavor of frustration until they finally realize that pleasing others all of the time is virtually impossible. People pleasing is a futile attempt to be all things to all people, and it only leads to stress. It is putting your happiness in the hands of someone else, depriving yourself of being in control of your own happiness. Eventually, caretakers must come to the realization that true acceptance comes from within.

Self-acceptance requires no standards. Learning to accept oneself with all one's limitations is true acceptance. People who accept you in the same manner are those who truly love you. Here is a caretaker's creed that I wrote for my students.

"I am lovable and capable. I am not perfect. I don't have to be. My worth cannot be measured by what others want me to be. The worth I have comes from the people in this world who love me for me— not for how I look or how I speak, but just for me.

I recognize that others also have worth. Life is not only about me. My purpose in life is to share my gifts and talents with others. My greatest feelings of accomplishment come from helping, not from getting. Through success and failure, I remain the same. I am lovable and capable. I have worth. I am accepted for who I am."

Loneliness

A devastating emotion that affects caretakers is *loneliness.* Ironically, a caretaker can be surrounded by people he or she cares for yet still feel extremely alone. The reason is that the people being cared for by the caretaker begin to take the caretaker for granted. They just expect the caretaker to always be there for them. They become so self-absorbed with their own needs that they fail to see that the caretaker also has needs that must be taken care of. They don't recognize the toll that is being taken on the person caring for them. It is as if all the love the caretaker gladly gives is never returned in kind.

Caretakers become lonely when they feel they have no one who can recognize and relate to their situation. They become frustrated at times when people don't recognize their needs. Deep inside, they become overwhelmed by the constant giving of themselves to others without receiving the same giving in return. They look for help and become frustrated when those they love and care for seem oblivious to their needs. They ask, "Why can't others see my needs?" or "Am I invisible?" or "Who takes care of the caretaker?" They begin to feel invisible. Standing up or speaking out for themselves, while healthy, is not in their comfort zone. It is in their DNA to give and not receive. Most of their outbursts from frustration are met with shock—and sometimes rejection.

Loneliness can lead to negative, unhealthy, or even paranoid thoughts in the mind of the caretaker. It can lead to a self-defeating sense of hopelessness and helplessness. It is a destroyer of self-worth. Caretakers suffering from loneliness may begin to feel that if they aren't caring for someone, they have no worth. Feelings of guilt and worthlessness may cause the caretaker to isolate himself or herself from others. Such caretakers don't feel worthy of being taken care of by others. They mistakenly see themselves as a bother to others if they have to ask for help in dealing with their own needs. Loneliness can also be directly related to depression and, in extreme cases, to suicide.

Frustration

Feelings of being upset or annoyed because of an inability to change or achieve something is known as *frustration*. Frustration occurs when one loses the ability to keep a realistic perspective on what one hopes will happen (expectations) and what can actually happen (reality).

The stress of being a caretaker can be very frustrating. Trying to constantly meet the needs of others is not an easy thing to do. The caretaker may begin to feel fatigued, used, and underappreciated. Frustration can lead to other emotions, such as anger and feelings of desperation. The feeling of being overlooked or invisible when it comes to somebody caring for them can exacerbate stress levels to an even higher state.

The caretaker must keep in mind that life is filled with ups and downs, so it is important to enjoy the good times, instead of just focusing on the bad. While life cannot be changed, how the caretaker allows life events to affect him or her can.

One way the caretaker can deal with frustration is by incorporating relaxation activities into their daily schedule. Nonstrenuous exercise, like going for a walk or a jog or doing yoga, can relax your muscles and make you feel calmer. More strenuous exercise can also help burn off frustration, allowing the caretaker to clear his or her mind of stress.

Truth about Emotions

Whatever the emotion that causes caretaker stress, the effects on health and relationships are very real. Here are some simple rules about emotions that may be helpful for caretakers:

Emotions are normal. They are neither positive nor negative. To feel happy, sad, excited, or mad is perfectly normal. Situations determine that your emotions will be based on what you are going through at the moment. To feel, even if it is to hurt, means you are alive. People who feel nothing are depressed. While emotions are neither good nor bad, how you express them may be. (See number three below.)

Feelings are not facts. They are temporary. Emotions are like the weather; they change. Today it may be cloudy. Tomorrow might be sunny. Just because you feel lousy today doesn't mean you *are* lousy or that you will feel lousy tomorrow. See your emotions as temporary feelings that can change at any time.

Expression is the opposite of depression. Finding healthy ways to express emotions is a key to good mental health. Holding emotions inside too long is not good. Suppressing emotions can lead to depression and other problems. Talk them out, cry them out, exercise them out, write them out—whatever is best for you, get them out. Once you get them out, you will relieve your stress.

The best way to deal with emotions is to begin by acknowledging they exist. Once an emotion is acknowledged, the caretaker must then identify what has caused it to exist. It is then up to the caretaker to find a way to express the emotion in a healthy way. What happens to a person is not nearly as important as the person's *reaction* to what happened. Seeing the big picture and maintaining a positive attitude can help the caretaker find ways of dealing with a wide range of emotions.

Below, make a list of emotions you deal with most often, along with healthy ways to express them instead of letting them build up inside of you.

_____
_____
_____
_____
_____
_____
_____
_____

Who Takes Care of the Caretaker?

CHAPTER 6
CARETAKERS AND PERSONALITY TYPES

People come with different personality types. Each causes different types of stress for the caretaker. Two types of personalities that caretakers deal with are Type A and Type B.

Type A personalities display competitiveness, drive, ambition, aggressiveness, and impatient behavior. They tend to see the world and others as something to conquer.

Type B personalities are more laid-back and flexible, and they are less rushed. They tend to enjoy life's experiences, rather than seeing the world as a competition.

Type A personalities cause more stress for the caretaker because they insist on ever-growing expectations for perfection. Type As are demanding, with little patience. There is no room for errors or mistakes. Type A personalities can be very aggressive in their communication with others, putting results ahead of feelings.

Type B personalities produce less stress for caretakers because of their laid-back pace. The frustration with Type B personalities comes from trying to get them to get anything done. They see no need to meet a deadline, preferring to procrastinate. They are constantly late for an appointment—if they remember to make one in the first place.

Constantly having to push Type B personalities to get them to do what they have to do is very stressful for the caretaker.

Beware of Narcissists

In 564 BC, the ancient Greek fabulist Aesop said, "Beware of wolves in sheep's clothing." When it comes to the caretaker's relationship with a narcissist, this advice still rings true.

Some people are by nature caretakers. They possess very dominant qualities of caring and nurturing. They see relationships as a service of love for another person. Like innocent sheep, caretakers can be very vulnerable to lurking danger.

A personality type that can be very dangerous for a caretaker to get involved with is the narcissist. A direct opposite of caretakers, narcissists lack empathy for others. Narcissists target and choose relationships based solely on how they can personally benefit, rather than on love. Things they look for in their targets are money, status, emotional support, or anything that can boost their childish egos.

Narcissists hide behind a mask when first meeting a caretaker. They may use an outgoing, sympathetic personality to lure caretakers into their trap. Once caught, the caretaker wakes up one day to find a whole different personality from the person they began to love and care for. It is very common to little by little discover a rude, mean, sadistic personality that was hiding behind the mask.

Caretakers are easy targets of abuse from narcissists, both verbally and physically. They are quick to put down or make fun of others to build up their own lack of self-esteem. A narcissist takes no responsibility for his or her actions. This type of person does not feel—or care how others feel.

Because this personality is so opposite their own, caretakers cannot understand what is happening. They have no concept of how someone can just use other people for selfish reasons. The caretaker, being driven by real love, often dismisses or makes excuses for the narcissist's behavior, hoping things will change. When relationships evolve to the point that narcissists can no longer get what they want from caretakers, they discard them like old shoes.

The caretaker is then left feeling confused, hurt, violated, and used. They wonder if the narcissist ever loved him or her. The answer is no. Narcissists love no one but themselves.

Once the relationship ends, the caretaker must begin the difficult task of rebuilding his or her own self-esteem, which has been severely damaged by the rejection and cruel behavior of the narcissist.

With counseling, caretakers eventually realize the emotional trap they have just escaped was not their fault. Healing begins when they finally realize they were deliberately targeted, lied to, and manipulated by the narcissist for their own gain. There was nothing they could have done differently. It is very important that the caretaker close the door on any and all future contact with the narcissist to prevent further emotional damage. If you are a caretaker, beware. The narcissistic wolf is out there lurking.

No problem is ever addressed until you become aware that it exists. While caring and serving others may be the dominant personality trait of the caretaker, learning to recognize, deal with, and in some cases avoid other personalities is essential to the well-being of a caring heart.

Take a moment to list below how different personality types affect you. Make a list of strategies you have found to be more effective for each type. Identifying each personality type and having a reaction strategy ready makes dealing with different personalities less stressful.

CHAPTER 7

THE ABCS OF COPING SKILLS FOR CARETAKERS

By definition, coping skills are methods a person uses to deal with stressful situations. Obtaining and maintaining good coping skills does take practice. However, utilizing these skills becomes easier over time. Most importantly, good coping skills make for good mental health and wellness.

The following is a list of twenty-six ways to cope with the stress of being a caretaker. They are not in any way designed to replace medical advice or prescribed treatment from a doctor. They are additional tools to help reduce, and in some cases eliminate, stress from this increasingly demanding world.

A. Avoid Perfectionism

When most people look in a mirror, they don't like what they see. They immediately focus on the flaws in their appearance that they would like to change. Others may not even notice, but for the person looking in the mirror, the flaws stand out. In other words, they don't see perfection.

Perfectionists are people who strive for flawlessness. They set excessively high performance standards accompanied by overly critical evaluations. Perfectionism is said to be the enemy of creativity—and ultimately of sanity. Trying to hold on to some unrealistic standard for yourself is tiring and stressful. The truth is that no one is perfect. All people have flaws. We are all prone to making mistakes at times.

As I write this book, as carefully as I try to word sentences, I know that editing and changes will be necessary. It is part of the process. If I got too hung up on making sure the manuscript was perfect the first time I wrote it, I would not get very far. Instead of a pleasurable adventure, it would turn into a painstakingly miserable task.

As a caretaker, you would not expect perfection in others, so stop expecting it in yourself. Break the stress of perfectionism. Give yourself a little room for editing in life. Remember, we are all works in progress; it is what makes us human. Maybe then you won't cringe so much the next time you look in the mirror.

B. Be Careful of Negative People
"You are who you hang out with" is an old saying that holds a lot of truth. If you want to be a positive, happy person, you have to distance yourself from negativity. It is one thing to vent frustrations with a friend at times, but some people thrive on always seeing things in a negative, sarcastic light. Understand that misery really does love company. Miserable people want those around them to be miserable as well. If you start to be more positive about life, don't be surprised if the doomsayers interject some form of skepticism toward your view. When things do go wrong, it reinforces their negative outlook. In a sense it becomes a self-fulfilling prophecy—a "See, I told you so!" mentality that cancels out all hope of optimism.

Being positive in a stressful world is not something that comes naturally. You actually have to work on it by developing coping skills to make yourself happy. One skill is to recognize the doom and gloom of negative people so that you don't get pulled in to their way of thinking. One way to counter the negativity of a miserable person you must be around is to say nice things. If that doesn't work, *say nice things really loudly* so that they get your message.

C. Create Space

One of the greatest stressors for caretakers caring for people is a lack of space. To give you a quick example of how lack of space affects your stress level, just go to a crowded mall at Christmastime, and then check your stress level when you leave. Too small an area filled with people increases tension levels.

All humans need a certain amount of personal space around them in order to feel comfortable. Here is a general rule to remember: the more stressed you are, the more space you need to decompress.

In my hometown there is a place in our city park called Lookout Point. It is a high hill where you can see the Missouri River bottoms for miles below. As kids we used to race from the bottom of the hill to the top. When we grew tired, we would sit on top of the hill and just stare at the scenery below. Looking at all that space gave me a strong sense of peace and tranquility. Even as an adult, I still enjoy going there when I feel stressed. It is a great place to go to "chill out."

Look for ways to create space in your life. If you are forced to exist in a crowded environment, put on a pair of headsets to create some personal space by losing yourself in enjoyable music. This goes for being around friends and loved ones as well. Sometimes, even if it is a person you love, you need to get away for a while to recharge your batteries.

As a caregiver, when you feel the walls crashing in, create space.

D. Don't Forget about Your Down Time

One of the greatest stressors for caretakers is time stress. Time stress is the feeling that you just don't have enough time to get everything done. Feeling overwhelmed by lack of time shouldn't be a surprise for a person dedicated to sacrificing their time for others. Realize that there are only so many hours in the day. You can only get so much done, and then it is time for a break.

Nobody is at his or her best when tired. Getting away from caretaking for a while sometimes leads to a whole new perspective on how to solve a problem when you return. Take a break. Take a nap. Go for a walk or a drive. Give yourself plenty of recovery time before you begin again.

Understand that for your own health the time away from caretaking is just as important as the time helping others. Your body and mind need a chance to recover. Denying yourself the opportunity to refresh eventually leads to burnout. Make sure you spend just as much time off for yourself as on tasks for others.

E. Exercise

Walking, jogging, sports, yoga, hobbies like reading, painting, writing, collecting, antiquing, beading, puzzles, and playing cards are all examples of healthy ways to get the blood flowing with fresh oxygen to the brain, taking your mind off your problems.

These types of activities allow you to escape stress for a while, so that you can recharge your physical and emotional batteries. Besides the obvious health benefits, fresh air and sunshine during a brisk walk outside can help you sort out the jumbled mess floating around in your head.

Spending time on games and hobbies distracts your thinking from your daily caretaking duties. Instead of worrying so much about others, spending some time doing something you find interesting fulfills the aesthetic needs described by Maslow. The sense of accomplishment one feels when completing one of these tasks can be exhilarating, leading to a sense of pride in oneself.

I know of some men who see mowing grass as a form of therapy. Whatever it is that works for you, my advice is to get up, get moving, or get interested in something other than your daily caretaking tasks.

F. Fun

Take time to enjoy comedy, music, and funny people. Psychiatrist Dr. Sidney Freedman, a character from the hit seventies TV show *MASH*, about a group of caretaking doctors and nurses helping wounded soldiers during the Korean War, once gave this advice about how to handle stress: "Ladies and gentlemen, take my advice. Pull down your pants, and slide on the ice."

An article from *Psychology Today* entitled, "Laughter: The Best Medicine," written by Hare Estroff Marano and published April 5, 2005, credits laughter with improving the flow of oxygen to the heart and brain, decreasing pain, improving job performance, and connecting people emotionally. Playwright and poet William Congreve wrote the famous line, "Music has charms to soothe a savage breast." Both have the capacity to reduce tension related to stress.

Whether it is finding a comedy club, watching a funny movie or TV show, or just hanging with people who make you laugh, there are many ways to lighten your mood and thus relieve your stress. Putting on a headset to listen to your favorite genres of music can have the same effect. Again, any type of distraction from your worries for others is therapeutic.

When my son is filled with worry and stress, one of my favorite things is to go to my computer and look up the dumbest jokes I can find. Then I start telling them to him. They are so painfully stupid that eventually he has to laugh.

The people able to handle the most stress in life are those with a good sense of humor.

G. Get Organized

Have a plan, stick to the plan, and always have a backup plan. Confusion is very stressful. It leads to a feeling that things are out of control. To avoid confusion it is important to develop a plan of attack. This feeling of direction brings a calming sense of order to chaos.

Once you have your plan, follow it. Constantly changing back and forth before you even see if your plan will work leads to doubt, confusion, and frustration. If you find that your plan is not working, *then* you can consider changing. But be careful; changing horses in the middle of the stream can lead to disastrous results.

Another bit of wisdom here is to always remember Murphy's Law, which says, "Anything that can go wrong will go wrong—at the most inopportune time." Life has a way of throwing curve balls from out of the blue. Having a backup plan will lead to a sense of calmness during hectic times. As a leader, your backup plan instills confidence in your mind that, no matter what happens, you have things under control.

H. Harbor Gratitude

The word *gratitude* comes from the Latin word *gratia*, meaning gratefulness. Gratitude is a feeling of thankfulness or appreciation. Gratitude helps the caretaker appreciate the good in life. It improves one's outlook when facing adversity, and it improves relationships as well.

It doesn't cost a penny to be thankful. Make a list of people for whom you are most thankful. The people on this list are those who give your face a smile. Never take the people on it for granted. Prioritize your life around those on your list.

I. Invest in Your Health

Have regular checkups. Stop ignoring symptoms. If you are hurting physically or emotionally, see your doctor. Don't disregard medications that are designed to help deal with stress. Follow the instructions on the prescriptions carefully and fully. If they don't work for you, call your doctor to make necessary adjustments.

Don't just give up on your health. Eat regularly. Stop skipping meals because you are too busy. Skipping meals only lowers your energy that you need to accomplish your caretaking of others effectively. You are only going to get out of your body what you put into it.

When young, we all have a tendency to take our health for granted. But as time passes, we come to the realization that this is not wise. Investing in your health will pay dividends in the long run. The other option—ignoring your health until a serious medical problem occurs—is a recipe for disaster.

J. Just Say No to More Commitments

A common complaint from caretakers who are too busy is that everybody wants something from them. People want them to join their group, committee, or organization. They are seen as a valuable asset.

The only problem is that every group, committee, or organization one joins requires a commitment of time and energy. This adds unnecessary demands to life, something that an already time-stretched person doesn't need.

No matter how worthwhile new commitments may seem, they are just adding more stress to your life. By not joining, the caretaker may feel some guilt at first, but in the long run, the caretaker is looking out for his or her own best interests. No one can blame you for that. Caretakers should think of themselves as their own booking agents, charged with protecting a valuable client. Making sure that they are rested, focused, and at their best for the important commitments in their life is important. It is easy to say yes, but the busier you are, the more you must say no.

K. Keep Moving Forward

There's no sense in crying over spilled milk. Stop beating yourself up over mistakes.

My grandfather was a house painter. In his lifetime, he must have painted hundreds of houses—inside and out. He was a happy, outgoing man who made friends easily. It wasn't hard to tell that he loved his work as well as his life. He was also an excellent painter. No one could paint a wall like Grandpa. Consequently, he was always in demand.

Once while I was in college, I went to help Grandpa paint a house. While working inside, I noticed how skilled he was at giving a wall a quality coat of paint so quickly. As a matter of fact, he could carry on a conversation with the homeowner, laughing all the time, while painting three walls to my one.

At one point he stopped to watch me. He noticed how I took my time dipping the brush in the paint bucket—and how I carefully wiped off both sides of the brush as I pulled it out, so as not to waste any paint. I then spread a thin coat of paint on the wall without spilling a drop. It was a slow, tedious process, but I dared not laugh or kid around for fear of making a mess.

Finally, Grandpa offered to give me some advice. "Here, watch this," he said, as he took the brush from my hand. Dipping the brush deep into the bucket, he produced a brush heaping with paint as he pulled it out. "See?" he said. "This is how you do it. Don't worry about spills and messes. They can always be cleaned up. Treat a wall the way you treat people—be generous. Have fun. Always put enough paint on the brush."

With that he turned and applied a thick coat of paint on the wall, while at the same time resuming his conversation with the homeowner. Yes, he did spill a few drops, but I noticed how much better his wall looked than mine. I also noticed how much fun he was having while painting it.

I've always remembered the lesson my grandfather taught me that day. Life is not always perfect. Some days we spill very few drops; some days we spill a lot. The only thing that really matters is what the wall looks like when we are done—and how much fun we had painting it. Don't live life in fear of mistakes. Put enough paint on your brush!

L. Live for the Moment

Quit worrying about what might happen. Worry is very fatiguing. Carrying around the weight of the world wears on one's emotional well-being. The Bible has some very sound advice when it comes to worry. Matthew 6:34 says, "Do not worry about tomorrow, for tomorrow will care for itself. Each day has enough trouble of its own."

Taking on the tasks of today is enough. Focus on one day at a time. Trying to add the weight of the future is just too overwhelming. It's much like chipping away at a rock and having the whole mountain fall on your head. Who needs that? Let tomorrow take care of itself. Face tomorrow when you are more rested. Today's worries really are enough for today.

M. Make a Difference in Someone Else's Life
Caretakers who become too stressed tend to isolate themselves from their friends. They become so consumed with their own responsibilities that they fail to recognize the therapeutic power of reaching out to others.

Be more friendly and generous to people. Seek out small ways to help others that don't take a lot of time or commitment. A caretaker friend of mine and I make a point every week to go out in the morning and play nine holes of golf. It only takes a couple of hours, but the therapeutic value is priceless.

When you meet new people, be the one to open communication lines. Be the first to say hello. Reach out to give a compliment. You will be surprised by what you receive in return.

Proverbs 12:25 says, "An anxious heart weighs a man down, but a kind word cheers him up." It only takes a moment to reach out to be a friend, but to the one who needs you, the memory never ends. Visiting with a friend, an elderly person, or a neighbor has a way of making one stop focusing on just oneself. The

Who Takes Care of the Caretaker?

attention you give and get from these interactions can help satisfy your emotional need for attention.

N. Never Underestimate Yourself

In many of my motivational speeches, I use the following affirmations: "People count. People matter. You count. You matter. You make a difference!" I have found it to be the most audience-captivating moment of the whole presentation.

Caretakers who are too stressed don't feel appreciated. Sometimes they feel like cogs in a machine used only to produce for others. Rarely are they told what an important impact they have on the ones they love. Sometimes they wonder if they really make a difference. This goes directly to what Maslow described as the need for self-actualization. In other words, people need to feel they have a purpose. They need to feel they are making a contribution to the greater good.

The simple fact is that we humans have the capacity to affect other human beings in ways we are never aware of until much later. I cannot tell you how many students have come up to me years after they left my class to tell me what a difference I made in their lives. At the time I had them in class, I didn't even know they were listening.

Caretakers believe their purpose in life is to use their gifts and talents to help others. That is truly the work of angels. As a caretaker, never underestimate your value to those around you. You do count! You do matter! You do make a difference!

O. Open Your Environment

As I mentioned before, the more stressed caretakers become, the more they may want to just find a cave to hide in. In fact, the opposite is what they need. One way to ease stress is to expand your surroundings to the outside world.

Many caretakers spend their days in a closed, controlled environment. Dark, dreary, and sterile. *Find a way to change that!* Open windows. Open blinds. Let the sun shine in. Breathe in the fresh air. If that is not possible, find ways to decorate your environment in light, bright colors. Hang posters of inspiring environmental scenes like beaches, mountains, or simply the sky. Add motivation or humor. Find motivational quotes that relate to you. Place them in locations you are sure to look at from time to time. Hang up cartoons or funny quips that make you smile.

Do whatever you can do to change your dreary cave into an environment of openness, tranquility, motivation, and fun.

P. Prioritize

Maybe under the letter *P*, I should have said, "Prozac," but instead I chose the word *prioritize*. Not everything has the same importance. Some demands are more pressing than others. Looking at all the tasks ahead of you can be very daunting, adding to your sense of time stress.

By definition, a *priority* is that which is regarded as more important than another. Instead of trying to handle everything that comes your way, it is important to prioritize that which is most important.

A number of years ago, as a classroom teacher, my teaching load was 136 students a day. I was also a husband and the father of a young son. As any caretaking parent with an elementary student knows, it is easy to be lured into serving on PTA committees, coaching youth sports, and teaching Sunday school. Loving my son so much, I wanted to do all I could to be involved in his life. But it was just too much.

What I quickly learned was that, while every activity was worthwhile, each one came with its own set of expectations and responsibilities, adding more stress to my already very busy schedule.

It wasn't long before I was stretched so thinly while trying to be all things to all people that I was just exhausted. The exhaustion led to stresses on the job and at home. All my relationships suffered as I began to see everyone as just another person who wanted something more from me.

I finally learned to prioritize what was really important to me. I discovered that it was more important to have time and energy to spend with my family and my main job of teaching my students. Some people may not have understood why I declined to get involved in their activities, but it was best for my son, my students, and myself.

I consciously made the decision that my son and students were my priorities. It was important for me to be at my best when nurturing them. While it was hard to say no to other commitments at first, eventually I saw that they would get along just fine without me.

Make a list of your responsibilities, ranking them in order from most important to least. Then see if there is anything on the list that can be eliminated or delegated to someone else. With the list that remains, try to make a conscience effort to decide how much time and energy you will spend with each priority. Remember, the most important priorities will take the most time. One important thing. *Do not forget to include time for rest and relaxation on your final priority list.* If you do, you will find fulfilling the rest of your priority list more and more difficult.

Q. Quit Trying to Be a Superhero

Ever feel like you have to be Superman in order to save everyone? Maybe you see yourself as a rescuer for those around you. You somehow feel the need to have a hand in everything, just to make sure everyone's taken care of.

Many caretakers are surprised by how people seem to go on just fine without them after they retire from their caretaking responsibilities. If only they had known, they might have spent a little less time sacrificing their entire lives in trying to be everything to everybody. Maybe they would have spent a little more time making lasting memories with the people they cared for. If only they had known. Well, now you know. You are a human *being*, not a human *doing*. Don't try to be a superhero.

R. Remain Positive

Out of the worst comes the best. Sometimes the brightest light comes from our darkest hours. History is full of examples in which people have done remarkable things during times of great hardship. The famous church hymn "Just as I Am, without One Plea" was written by Charlotte Elliott, an invalid who suffered greatly for most of her last fifty years of life. She somehow found it in her heart to write words that will be sung by churchgoers until the end of time.

Vincent van Gogh only sold one painting in his lifetime, and that was to a friend for a small amount of money. Still, he continued to paint, even while starving at times, accumulating some eight hundred works. Today, his paintings bring in millions. Remaining positive in the face of adversity requires patience and perseverance. Both qualities are essential when dealing with caretaking in stressful situations. Stay positive.

S. Slow Down

John Wooden, the famous basketball coaching legend from UCLA, would tell his players, "Be quick, but don't rush." It's good advice for all of us. Feeling rushed and overwhelmed is very stressful.

During times of high stress, make a concerted effort to slow yourself down. Walk more slowly. Take a deep breath. If you come across something interesting or inspiring, come to a stop to soak it in. Let things come to you for a change, instead of always chasing after them. If you feel yourself becoming anxious or irritable from too many demands coming at you all at once, repeat the following: *Slow down. Don't get frustrated. Focus on one thing at a time.*

There is an old song sung by Mac Davis entitled "Stop and Smell the Roses." The words of the song offer some good advice. Here are a few lines:

> Hey Mister, where you going in such a hurry?
> Don't you think it's time you realized
> there's a whole lot more to life than work and worry?
> The sweetest things in life are free
> and they're right before your eyes.
>
> Chorus:
> You've got to stop and smell the roses.
> You've got to count your many blessings every day.
> You're going to find your way to heaven is a rough and rocky road
> If you don't stop and smell the roses along the way.

Remember, you can't enjoy what you don't take time to notice. Slow down.

T. Try New Things

Expand your horizons. Sometimes in your caretaking, it is easy to get stuck in a rut. Have you ever tried something new, only to discover that you really like it? It's like "Wow, this is different, new—fun!" Sometimes we get so tied to our normal routines that our existence becomes stale. Boredom sets in. Believe me, there is nothing worse than being bored. Spend long hours waiting in airports if you want to know how stressful boredom can become. The British poet William Cowper wrote a long time ago that "Variety is the spice of life." So true.

If you find your daily routine is getting a little stale, look for ways to spice things up a bit. The same is true for your life in general. You don't have to totally discard the tried and true routines of the past, but don't fear at least looking at ways to make things a little new or different. Spice up your life. Look for variety.

U. Understand Your Sensitivities

Self-reflection is helpful for caretakers in dealing with stress. Knowing what your stressors are is important. Things that really get you going may not affect the next person the same way. You are different from everyone else. Understanding what annoys you helps you to plan ahead to avoid pitfalls before they happen. Developing coping skills allows you to stop stress before it starts to build up.

Understand how you communicate with others. Being too passive allows things to build up inside until you act out, sometimes in a negative way. Being too aggressive causes hurt feelings in other people, causing tension among peers. Try to be assertive in standing up for yourself. Only you can know those things that bother you the most.

V. Voice Your Thoughts and Opinions

There is a saying that expression is the opposite of depression. People who don't express—or who don't feel worthy enough to express—eventually become depressed. It is very frustrating to never be asked your opinion.

Imagine being a loyal, productive employee for many years who has taken pride in your work to make the company successful. Then a new boss comes along and changes everything. You are never consulted. Someone higher up who has no experience thinks he has a better way for you to do your job. That would be frustrating.

Your emotional needs of feeling valued and recognized for your efforts are ignored. You need to find a way to vent, so you go home and dump it all on your spouse. Even though your spouse has no clue about half the things you are venting about, it still feels good to talk to somebody. Getting all that frustration out instead of bottling it up inside relieves stress. I tell people it is kind of like throwing up. It may not be pretty when it comes out, but it sure makes you feel much better once it is gone.

W. Who Is in Control?

Feeling that life is out of control is very stressful. As human beings we long for a sense of order in our lives. Unless you are a very creative person, chaos is stressful.

We need always to keep in mind that we are in charge of our careers; our careers are not in charge of us. Take some ownership in learning to control the demands being heaped upon you by others at work. Make a conscious effort to look for ways to make your job more manageable. Set some limits. Stick to them as much as possible. See your work as a way to fulfill your needs, not as something you constantly sacrifice for. Be in charge. Be assertive. Take control.

X. Extra Care and Attention for You

Caretakers don't want pity. No one wants to be seen as needy. Everyone needs to be able to address their needs, just like anybody else. The more stressed you

Who Takes Care of the Caretaker?

become the more you need to focus on caring for yourself.

Taking a long hot bath, getting a massage, or sleeping in are all examples of taking a little extra care and attention for yourself. Don't look at it as being needy but rather as a necessity for someone as busy as you are. It is not selfish to care for yourself. You are no good to others or to your job if you are burnt out.

Plan special times in your busy schedule just for you. Don't feel guilty. You are worth it!

Y. You Can Do It! Give Yourself a Pep Talk!

We all engage in "self-talk." It is a way of affirming ourselves in a positive or negative manner. When we're too stressed, it is easy to get negative with ourselves as well as with the world around us. We may even get down on ourselves for getting into this stressful mess. We get down on others for not recognizing our needs or rescuing us. Either way, the negativity deletes whatever precious energy we have left, emotionally and physically, from caring for others.

Believe it or not, being more positive in our self-talk helps. Giving yourself a pat on the back through words of encouragement is a way of recognizing your own self-worth. Recognize that no one is perfect, but you are doing a good job. You should be proud of your efforts as well as your accomplishments. If nobody around you takes time to recognize you, recognize yourself.

Every team needs a cheerleader. You deserve one as well. Remind yourself constantly of your own self-worth.

Z. Find Your Zest for Life

What do you like to do? Where would you like to go? What are you really interested in? Sometimes we all get so caught up with things we have to do in our daily routines that we start to ignore the things we like to do. The things we like are what add motivation to our day. It is a little easier making it through a busy work week if you know there is a dream vacation coming the next week. Looking forward brings optimism.

Always remember, the greatest song ever written, the greatest painting ever painted, the greatest invention ever invented, and the greatest athletic feat ever accomplished were all done by people who wanted to do them—not people who *had* to do them. They were motivated by what they liked, loved, or were interested in doing. We all have things in life we have to do, but spending time on what we *like* to do brings a zest for living.

CONCLUSION

Caretakers are wonderful people. I consider them the salt of the earth. They are givers of themselves to others, nurturing those around them. But they are only human. Because of their nature, they are very susceptible to stress—stress that leads to fatigue, causing feelings of frustration, isolation, guilt, and doubt. Because they are caretakers of others, they tend to focus solely on others, to the detriment of themselves.

The fact is that caretakers also have needs that should be met. Even the greatest caretaker of all time, Jesus of Nazareth, needed to be alone at times for rest, restoration, and reflection. This question is reflected in the title of this book: *Who takes care of the caretaker?*

This book defined both who caretakers are and how the stress of being a caretaker affects one's physical and mental health. It pointed out a specific type of stress—chronic stress—which causes many caretakers to suffer from the debilitating effects of chronic fatigue. Other common effects too much stress can have on a caretaker's emotional health were also listed. We looked at how different personality types can affect a caretaker's stress. Finally, twenty-six coping skills were listed that caretakers can use to reduce their stress.

"Who takes care of the caretaker?" seems like a question that should not have to be asked. Everyone should recognize and value the caretakers in their lives. We all should show our thankfulness to these loving people who play such a nurturing role for us, and we should return the favor by showing care for them. Unfortunately, that doesn't always happen. Sadly, many caretakers are left alone to care for themselves.

Reading this book to understand the problems stress can cause on a caretaker's health is one thing, but doing something about it is another. In order for you, the caretaker, to face the changes needed to reduce stress, there is one more word I must write about: *courage.*

Who Takes Care of the Caretaker?

One of the most misunderstood virtues in life is courage. Many people wrongly believe that, because they have fear, they somehow lack courage. In fact courage cannot exist without fear. If you are not afraid to do something, it takes no courage to do it. It is only when you are scared to death that you understand the true meaning of courage. *Courage is having the guts to keep trying, even when you know you could lose.*

I remember watching a group of young children taking swimming lessons as they jumped off the diving board for the first time. Some of the children had no trouble running and jumping into the deep water. Other children could not bring themselves to do it. One little boy stood on the end of the board and cried because he was afraid. Finally, with the instructor's encouragement, he gathered his courage and jumped. All of the parents who were watching from the side of the pool cheered the young boy as he swam to the ladder. The little boy learned a lesson about courage that day.

It takes courage for any great changes in life to occur. For caretakers, changing their reactions to the stressful world around them will not be easy. They may feel afraid of what could happen. It will take conscious effort on their part to face the fear and jump into their future. Recognition of a problem is only part of the solution. To solve a problem, one must face the problem and fix it. *We all have issues. We live with our issues until they cause us conflict. Then we deal with them. If we fail to deal with our issues, we live with the consequences.*

Only when caretakers take the time to truly understand the toll their caretaking has on their health—and then act differently—will things change. Until then they will continue marching to the beat of frustration and fatigue, never truly finding the happiness they seek or the satisfaction in life they deserve.

Okay. Enough information and advice. Now, what are you going to do?

Remember this: People count; people matter. You count; you matter. As a caretaker, you make a difference in the lives of people around you. Now, go out and do the same for yourself. Be good to yourself. You deserve it. *You take care of the caretaker!*

ABOUT THE AUTHOR

Tom Krause received his master's in education from the University of Missouri–Columbia in 1988. He is the author of *Touching Hearts, Teaching Greatness*, *The Little Boy's Smile*, *A Teen's Guide to Not Being Perfect*, and *Go Big Blue: The Story of the 1974 Boonville Pirates*. He is a contributing author to many books in the Chicken Soup for the Soul series. His additional writings have appeared in many publications around the world.

As an international inspirational speaker, Tom presents for hundreds of clients nationwide and overseas in the fields of education, volunteerism, and business. His "You Make a Difference!" presentation consistently receives standing ovations as audiences spontaneously react to Tom's inspiring message. Tom's presentations empower people to success and happiness in life using three principles he has taught for over thirty years: *Be yourself. Believe in yourself. Don't be afraid to go for your dreams*! Tom is considered one of America's most-quoted inspirational speakers, and his motivational quotes appear in publications and on the Internet worldwide.

After thirty-one years of teaching health and coaching football in the Missouri Public School System, Tom retired in 2010. It has been estimated that nearly eight thousand students went through his classroom. He loved them all.

Contact Tom Krause at www.coachkrause.com.